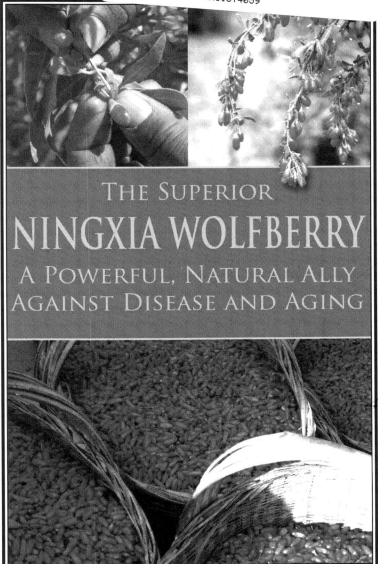

The Superior
NINGXIA WOLFBERRY
A Powerful, Natural Ally
Against Disease and Aging

The Superior Ningxia Wolfberry
A Powerful, Natural Ally Against Disease and Aging

For additional copies of this booklet please call:
1-800-524-4195 or visit www.yglgtools.com

TABLE OF CONTENTS

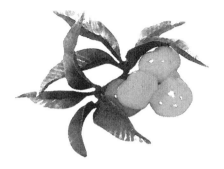

While wolfberry can grow in many different locations, it is important to understand that the research found in this booklet was conducted on wolfberry (Lycium barbarum), which originated in Ningxia, China. Although there are actually 17 different species of wolfberries, the Ningxia wolfberry is the most nutritionally dense, and the most researched and tested wolfberry on the market.

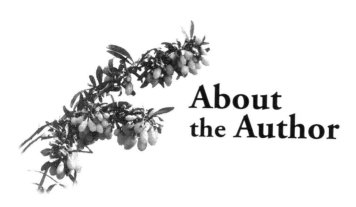

About the Author

Dr. Hugo Rodier, M.D., has a medical practice in Salt Lake City, Utah, and is a recognized authority in nutritional and integrative medicine and psycho-neural immunology.

Dr. Rodier has traveled the world, volunteering at clinics for displaced people and also in the National Health Service Corps. He studied at the Baylor College of medicine and the University of Utah Medical School.

He serves an active role as a member of the editorial board of the Utah Medical Association, he teaches at the University of Utah, and he is also chairman of the Utah Medical Association's Environmental Committee.

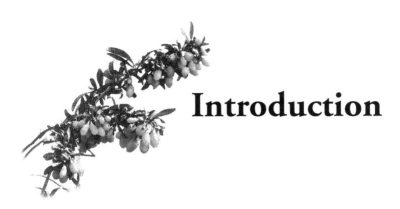

Introduction

The Ningxia wolfberry is a native Chinese vine adorned with trumpet-shaped flowers and deep red fruits. Known by ancients as the herb of transcendence, wolfberry has grown in Ningxia, China for hundreds of years and its fruit is highly valued for its pleasant taste, nutrient value and medicinal properties. A two-week festival celebrating wolfberry is held in Ningxia each year and draws worldwide attention to this regional specialty.

Wolfberry dates back to 25-220 AD. There are legends about the fruit dating back 5,000 years. The great healer, Shen Nung included wolfberry in the world's first pharmacopoeia, printed about 475 BC. A physician's handbook, Ben Zao Gen Mo, from the Ming dynasty also documents the use of wolfberry.

Highly regarded in China for centuries as one of its foremost nutritional and therapeutic plants, the Chinese wolfberry, crowned as the "red diamond," can be found in many ancient medical books.

Medicinally, wolfberry has been used to strengthen muscles and bone and stimulate tissue development. Wolfberry also improves liver function, restores vitality and improves vision. Wolfberry polysaccharides can enhance immunity, strengthen the immune system and can help prolong life. Scientists believe that wolfberry has strong anti-tumor properties and exerts anticancer effects.

Although wolfberry has been used in the Orient for thousands of years, its introduction to the United States is a more recent phenomenon. Gary Young documented the first use of wolfberry in the USA in 1996. Now his company is the largest importer of Ningxia Wolfberries in the USA. A greater distribution of quality Ningxia wolfberry products into America couldn't be timelier. There is a chronic problem overwhelming our society. Both patients and doctors have been indoctrinated to quickly reach for a drug that only treats the symptoms of problems, not the roots. The whole health care system is failing because we continue to apply acute care solutions, that is, pharmaceutical and surgical solutions to chronic problems that would be best approached by changing our lifestyles, and particularly our diets.

"It is essential that practicing physicians develop a working knowledge of herbs and stay abreast of these emerging findings in order to best advise their patients on the value of health promoting diets in disease and prevention... These are heady days for nutritional scientists as newer understandings of food and health promise to bring clinical nutrition to the forefront of clinical medicine. Practitioners must become nutritionally educated and oriented if they are to maintain their patients' confidence and stay abreast of this aspect of continuously evolving modern medicine."

("Nutrition Guidance of Family Doctors Towards Best Practice," Proceedings of the Third Heelsum International Workshop, Netherlands, December 2001; American Journal of Clinical Nutrition 2003;77:1001S).

These are indeed heady days, when everything we have intuited about health, disease and nutrition is being corroborated by very good science. This is causing a major shift in the way physicians address chronic issues of health and disease. Of course, naturopaths, chiropractors, herbologists and other care-givers have known that food is the best medicine from the get-go. So why have physicians mostly ignored nutrition in their practices, and have instead over-emphasized a pharmaceutical approach? It would be very easy to blame doctors. In fact, most people do. While physicians are likely part of the problem, we must look at less simplistic answers to this question.

Fortune Magazine has a more satisfactory explanation: *"We hate big pharma but we sure love drugs."* The Center for Disease Control reported that 44% of Americans are taking at least one drug and that 17% take three or more. Why? Because that is what most people want from doctors.

The education of doctors is largely influenced by pharmaceutical companies, which have made it all too easy for everyone to "sweep dirt under the carpet." In other words, we are all facilitating or enabling this reliance on the pharmaceutical approach. HMOs must share some of the responsibility for this system, too. Their "perverse incentives" have made it so that it is more rewarding to give people a quick prescription, rather than spend the time addressing the real issues, the real roots of our diseases. In other words, the molecular dys-equilibrium created by years of kilograms of poor nutrition is now addressed by a few milligrams of a drug that often has many adverse side effects.

So what can be done to address the chronic problems that are overwhelming our society? The answer to this question is urgently needed, since our society is rapidly aging. Soon baby boomers will overwhelm our health care system unless we make some drastic changes. Real answers are likely to test our political will and our economic reserves. Perhaps we are not ready as a society to strike at the root of the problems. Most people feel that the "patch" approach of half-way fixes in health care is here to stay, since only few are willing to tackle the problem head on.

I suggest we take the matter in our own hands and begin to make changes in our own lives and that of our loved ones by educating our friends, clients and patients. The simplicity of the answer is staggering. The *Journal of Science* tells us that "complexity" in health is a result of not understanding the simple principles underlying all conditions. This means that a "complex" health problem does not necessarily need complex solutions. Occam's razor, a Physics principle, tells us that whenever one is faced with many complex answers, the simplest is probably the correct one. So, what is this simple answer?

> *"Food is the best medicine,"*
> Hippocrates, father of ancient medicine.
> Maimonides, middle ages physician.
> Sir William Osler, father of modern medicine.

First, we need to change people's diet, which most of the time means making people aware of their refined sugar addiction. If people start eating the Mediterranean diet, which is full of the nutrients mentioned above, healing is noted in about 80% of problems very soon. Foods dense in antioxidants and anti-inflammatory micronutrients accelerate this process. This is why fruits and vegetables in general, and Ningxia wolfberry juice in particular are such beneficial agents. Specifically, wolfberry has been found to be very high in these micronutrients, which explains why wolfberry seems to help so many conditions; it can help repair the cell membranes by reducing oxidation, inflammation, toxicity and mitochondrial dysfunction.

Wolfberry also has an abundance of the right natural sugars that are essential to build sound glycoproteins that make up cell membrane receptors and cell messengers of communication. Digestive enzymes, particularly those in fruit juices like wolfberry, are mostly based on sugar. But these are the correct sugars needed for glycosylation of proteins. Digestive enzymes are powerful anti-inflammatory agents because they provide the right sugars for glycosylation of the cell membrane, thus reducing the inflammation of the membrane. *"Glycobiologists are more confident that a spoonful of sugar will not only make the medicine go down, but replace it with something that works better."*

These natural sugars, or saccharides from plants, can be absorbed directly into our bodies. Some still think that all sugars are broken down then rebuilt into needed sugars in the cell, but there is evidence that these basic sugars may be absorbed directly. Attaching the right sugars can help create new and more powerful drugs.

Occasionally, toxic microorganisms need to be removed form the intestines, where most of the immune system is found. Of course, the nutrients above are also healing the cell membranes lining the G.I. tract, thereby healing the immune system to better fight nox-

7

ious organisms. By doing so, we also improve absorption of the nutrients we ingest.

Secondly, we need to make sure these nutrients are being processed adequately. Most people start to lose digestive enzymes past the age of 40, so, supplementing them will also improve the absorption of these micronutrients. Digestive enzymes may be supplemented in various forms, including capsules and pills. Interestingly, fruits in general and wolfberry in particular are very high in natural digestive enzymes. It should also be pointed out that digestive enzymes have an anti-inflammatory and antioxidant effect.

Thirdly, we need to supplement probiotics or friendly organisms in the intestines to fight noxious organisms, reduce inflammation in the lining of the intestines, and in general improve the function of the immune system in the intestines. Probiotics need good food, particularly fiber to thrive. The Mediterranean diet provides higher amounts of fiber. Fruits and vegetables have 2-8 times more fiber than grains. Again, wolfberry helps by providing nourishment, especially fiber, to these benign organisms.

Is it truly as simple as the *Journal of Science* tells us? Modern research says yes, and so do I. The most powerful tool I have in my medical kit is my relationship with patients and their efforts to eat better and repair their cell membranes.

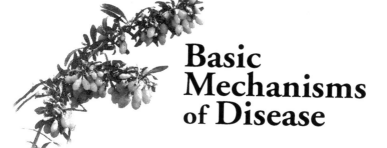

Basic Mechanisms of Disease

"Medicine will one day come to understand that there are very few principles underlying all health conditions. This is what we have discovered ourselves in Physics."

— David Deutch, Fabric of Reality.

Before discussing the many and wide variety of well-studied benefits of wolfberry, we must understand the basic mechanisms of health and disease. Then it will be extremely simple to see why the Ningxia wolfberry is so effective for practically all conditions and organ systems.

Let us start with a landmark article published in the *Journal of the American Medical Association 2004*; 291:358. It is titled "Neuroprotection in Parkinson's Disease," but it covers what many other journals are reporting to be the roots of all diseases. Basically, the authors tell us that the reason why cell membranes are becoming resistant to ALL messengers of communication, not just insulin, is because cell membranes are:

1. Inflamed
2. Oxidized
3. Toxic
4. Lacking in mitochondrial function to energize receptors to open and close

Cell membranes become more rigid and inflexible because of these mechanisms, thus less responsive to any cell messenger, not just insulin. And, why is this happening? Because we are lacking antioxidants, anti-inflammatory molecules, and micronutrients to fuel the mitochondria (energy furnaces of cells) and detoxification pathways of the Liver.

It starts in the cells and then begins to affect the entire body system. This is why we don't live as long and have more diseases when these basic mechanisms are not functioning properly. Some people attribute longevity and lack of disease to "good genes." While genetics is obviously a factor, 80 percent of diseases are linked to environmental and lifestyle issues. This was demonstrated by a study of 44,000 pairs of separated twins in Scandinavian countries.

And why such a lack of good micronutrients? We are not eating very good diets. The environment is so toxic that we burn up more antioxidants and anti-inflammatory molecules in our constant efforts to detoxify toxins that enter our bodies on a daily basis. Stress from poor relationships (human and environmental) also burns up these micronutrients. Soils are not as saturated with micronutrients as they used to be. So we end up with sub-optimal levels of these nutrients to build and fuel the optimal function of our cell membranes and our Psycho-Neuro-Immune-Endocrine system of cell communication.

We end up with poor tissue function as well. The weakened cell membranes that compose practically every tissue and organ of our bodies trigger significant dysfunction in the "terrain." Tissues like the intestines, lungs, skin, blood vessels, the brain, kidneys, etc., become "leaky." Why? Because of the four basic mechanisms outlined above. With those changes in every other organ, it is easy to see how disease will begin to manifest itself.

By now you are likely to see quite clearly why nutrition is going to prevent and heal so many conditions! And you will see the evidence provided by science to sustain us in our endeavors to make *"food the best medicine."*

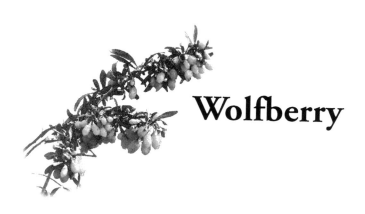

Wolfberry

Now that we have reviewed these basic principles of health and disease, we are ready to understand why wolfberry is so effective. Some find the range of benefits hard to believe. This is a sure sign they are focused on a pharmaceutical approach and do not understand the simple principles reviewed above. Also, it shows they are laboring under the worn-out philosophy of "one disease-one answer," which is nothing but a symptomatic approach to health care. This is the main reason our system of health care is so dysfunctional. What we must do is strike at the common root of health problems, then, *all of them will improve.*

Then there is the mater of EVIDENCE. You will see that wolfberry enjoys a wide and far-reaching bibliography to document its effectiveness. Of course the evidence is all along the lines of working on cell communication through the maximization of anti-oxidation, anti-inflammation, mitochondrial function, and detoxification. All this is achieved through a natural, whole food approach, instead of supplementation with artificial laboratory antioxidants. There is considerable evidence favoring the use of whole foods as sources of antioxidants. As you will see, this approach is much more scientifically valid.

Origins

The Ningxia wolfberry (Lycium barbarum) originated in Ningxia, China, where it is grown with organic farming techniques. Many wolfberry supplements are dried before they are imported into the United States. To insure the best results from this Chinese fruit it is important to find a company that imports a fresh wolfberry puree. This raw material insures that the natural healing agents found in the plant's juice, peel and flesh are present and intact.

The best berries are documented to grow in the Ningji Yi Hao County. Wolfberry imported from this area comes with a Green Food Certificate, guaranteeing that no fertilizers or pesticides have been used, nor sulfur, irradiation or dyes. There are no heavy metals (lead, arson, mercury, cadmium) in the Ningxia wolfberry.

The Yellow River runs through Ningxia and is used for irrigation. This river is well-known for its fertile silt deposits, which are rich in minerals. The farms in Ningxia are in a semi-arid region with plenty of sunlight and a high temperature difference between day and night. These conditions have earned Ningxia the distinction of being China's recognized "herbal medicine valley," assuring wolfberry's high nutritional contents and natural organic sugar accumulation.

This is why Ningxia has been named China's only medicinal wolfberry production base. Today, wolfberry is regarded as an important Chinese medicinal plant by the Institute of Genetics at the Academia Sinica in Beijing. Olympic Chinese coaches consider the Ningxia wolfberry their "secret weapon."

Basic Research on the Wolfberry

As established above, any product, whether pharmaceutical, synthetic vitamins, or whole foods, must work through the cell membrane of cells and its network of messengers. If the cell membrane is oxidized, inflamed, toxic or lacking in energy from the mitochondria, cell communication will break down, with dire consequences for the normal functioning of our bodies and minds.

So, logic dictates that Wolfberry must be working through these simple concepts to exert its well-documented benefits. Indeed.

The Brunswick oxygen radical absorbance capacity (ORAC) assay, a universally-known test for antioxidant and anti-inflammatory activity in foods has consistently ranked wolfberry as the food with the highest activity in these areas. The ORAC was developed by Tuft University. Free radicals, or Reactive Oxygen Species (ROS), cause oxidation, inflammation, toxicity and mitochondrial dysfunction in our bodies. There are several ROS produced by our metabolism and toxic environments, and foods can be tested to assay their capacity to neutralize these ROS.

Initials	Full name	Target ROS
ORAC	Oxygen radical absorbance capacity	Peroxyl
H-ORAC	Hydroxyl radical absorbance capacity	Hydroxyl
N-ORAC	Peroxynitrate radical absorbance capacity	Peroxynitrate
S-ORAC	Superoxide radical absorbance capacity	Superoxide

Since ROS cause cell membrane dysfunction as noted above, foods that counteract and neutralize ROS are going to strike at the very root of problems. Consequently, foods with the highest ORAC values have consistently shown to be of benefit in practically all conditions. Such is the case with wolfberry.

Ningxia wolfberry contains the highest natural amounts of important and rare antioxidants and sugars. The wolfberry grown on the Yellow River in the Ningxia province of China has the highest levels of immune-stimulating polysaccharides. The wolfberry found in this region is one of the most nutrient-dense foods, rich in many vitamins and minerals. Antioxidants such as those found in this berry are absolutely essential for life.

Wolfberry Ingredients

Before reviewing the evidence favoring wolfberry, we need to list the ingredients, or micronutrients found in wolfberry:

Polysaccharides: healthy sugars needed for cell membrane function and structure.

Polyphenols: they include flavones (like carotenoids,) isoflavones (genistein, deidstein, etc,) catechins (like green tea,) quercetin, proanthocyanidins (like grape seed extract,) galloylated tea, ellagic acid, and anthocyanidins.

Zeathanthin esters: antioxidants in wolfberry, other berries and several herbs.

Betaine: micronutrient indispensable for liver function, digestion, DNA function. Also very important in B-complex metabolism. Betaine is also found in wheat germ, spinach, beets, shrimp, and pretzels.

 16

Vitamin C: wolfberry has the highest content of vitamin C of all fruits and vegetables. It contains 148 mg/100mg, according to the USDA, 1999. Other foods, such as parsley spinach and cruciferous vegetables contain from 133 mg/100/mg to 93 mg. Oranges have 53 mg and tomatoes have 19 mg.

Calcium: wolfberry has 110 mg/100 mg, compared to 107 mg in Taro leaves. Cruciferous vegetables have about 50 mg, and cherries 16 mg (USDA 1999).

Beta carotene: wolfberry has 12,600 IU/100 gm, compared to 12,100 in chicken liver, 11,000 in carrots and 2,500 in apricots.

Fiber: four ounces of wolfberry contain 215 mg of fiber. Other antioxidants: beta-sitosterol, withanolides, P-coumaric acid, pyrroles, cerebrosides, lutein, cyclic peptides, acyclic diterpene glycosides, biotin, B vitamins, trace minerals, amino acids, and lyciumins.

Ningxia Wolfberry Juice

When looking for a product make sure it is made with a Ningxia wolfberry puree so that it contains the whole fruit in the product. A synergistic juice blend will further enrich its salutary affects. Look for a juice blend that contains Ningxia wolfberry, in addition to blueberry, pomegranate and raspberry juices, and lemon and orange essentials oils. This will give the juice an antioxidant spectrum with a high ORAC value.

The **pomegranate** represented life and regeneration in ancient Greece. In Buddhism, it is one of 3 blessed fruits. Three Royal

Colleges in England feature the pomegranate in their coats of arms. The National Institute of Cancer has reported on *"the extraordinary medicinal properties of the tree, an idea that dates to Biblical times and which has oddly been overlooked by Western medicine"* (J. National Cancer Institute 2003;95:346). Pomegranate has three times the antioxidant activity of green tea, or red wine. It reduces cholesterol by 40%.

Blueberry juice is also rich in proanthocyanidins. Tuft University studies have shown that it protects blood cells against free radical oxidation, and slows brain aging. Studies at Mainz University show that it protects cell DNA.

Raspberry juice has high levels of Ellagic acid, a polyphenol also found in wolfberry. Ellagic acid has become known for its anti-carcinogenic/anti-mutagenic effects. These traits help inhibit the growth of tumors and reduce the incidence of cancer. Ellagic acid is also known for its anti-bacterial and anti-viral properties.

Lemon and orange essential oils, like limonene, help combat cell mutations and increase glutathione levels in the liver. Glutathione is the end-product of all antioxidants.

As expected, wolfberry juice has a much higher ORAC value than other related juices; it has nearly three times the value of other leading juice blends.

The related H-ORAC, N-ORAC, and S-ORAC of wolfberry juice are also significantly higher than other brands listed.

RESEARCH EVIDENCE FOR THIS CHAPTER

Here is the research that shows wolfberry's high micronutrient contents decrease ROS and thus keep our cell membranes and our system of cell communication operational by keeping oxidation, inflammation, toxicity and mitochondrial dysfunction down to a minimum:

- "Scavenger capacity of Wolfberry crops on Superoxide radicals, Hydrogen peroxide, Hydroxyl radicals and Singlet oxygen," J. Agricultural Food Chemistry 2000;48:5677.
- "Scavenging effect of total flavonoids of Lycium barbarum on active oxygen radicals," J. Wei Sheng Yan Jiu 1998;27:109.
- "Identification and quantification of Zeaxanthin esters in plants (Lycium barbarum)," J. agricultural Food Chemistry 2003;51:7044.
- "Hepatoprotective (Liver) Pyrrole derivatives of Lycium chinese fruits," J. Bioorganic Medical Chemistry Letters 203;13:79.
- "Glycans (good sugars) isolated from the fruit of Lycium barbarum," J. Asian Natural Products Research 1999;1:259.
- "Structural features of arabinogalactan-proteins (good sugars) from the fruit of Lycium barbarum," J. Carbohydrate Research 2001;333:79.
- "Alpha tocopherol (vitamin E) content in tropical plants (Lycium,)" J. agricultural Food Chemistry 2001;49:3101.
- "Determination of Betaine in Lycium," J. Chromatography A 1999;857:331.
- "New antihepatotoxic Cerebroside from Lycium," J. Natural Products 1997;60:274.
- "Cyclic peptides, Acyclic diterpene glycosides in Lycium," J. Chemistry Pharmacology Bulletin 1993;41:703.
- "Zeaxanthin and Lutein pigments of Lycium," J. Annals Super Sanita 1969;5:51.
- "The protective effects of total falvonoids from Lycium on lipid peroxidation of Liver mitochondria," J. Wei Sheng Yan Jiu 1999;28:115.
- "Determination of four fractions of Lycium polysaccharides," J. Zhong Yao Cai 2001;24:107.
- "Physico-chemical properties and activity of glycoconjugate LbGp2 from lyceum barbarum," J. Yao Xue Bao 2001;36:599.
- "Inhibiting effects of Lycium barbarum polysaccharide on nonenzyme glycation," J. Biomedical Environmental Science 2003;16:267.
- "Effect of Lycium on defending free radicals of mice caused by hypoxia (lack of oxygen,)" J. Wei Sheng Yan Jiu 2002;31:30.
- "Effect of Wolfberry on DNA synthesis of the aging-youth 2BS fusion cells," J. Zhongguo Zhong Xi Yi Jie He Za Zhi 2003;23:926.

- "Studies on chemical constituents in fruit of Lycium barbarum," J. Zhongguo Zhong Yao Za Zhi 2001;26:323.
- "Experimental research on the role of Lycium barbarum polysaccharide in anti-peroxidation," J. Zhongguo Zhong Yao Za Zhi 1993;18:110.
- "Effect of Fructus Lycii on Mitochondrial DNA deletion, respiratory chain complexes and ATP synthesis in aged rats," J. Zhongguo Zhong Yao Za Zhi 2001;21:437.
- "Anti-inflammatory effects of Fructus Lycii," J. Ethnopharmacology 2003;89:139.
- "A polysaccharide-protein complex from Lycium barbarum upregulates cytokine expression in human peripheral blood mononuclear cells," European J. Pharmacology 2003;27:217.
- "Isolation and purification of Lycium barbarum polysaccharide and its antifatigue effect," J. Wei Sheng Yan Jiu 2000;29:115.

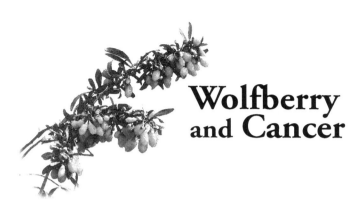

Wolfberry
and Cancer

It has been amply demonstrated that good nutrition will decrease the risk of cancer and prolong longevity. This is achieved by keeping our cell membranes and its network of communication healthy, flexible and well stocked with antioxidants and anti-inflammatory micronutrients. Even supplementation with these micronutrients helps. However, it is best to get them from whole, natural nutrients, such as the wolfberry. As shown above, wolfberry has the highest natural amounts of certain health-promoting antioxidants and good sugars of any food (more evidence below,) including synthetic antioxidant supplementation:

The key question is whether a purified phytochemical has the same health benefits as does the whole food. Our group found that the vitamin C in apples with skin accounts for only .4% of the total antioxidant activity. We propose that the additive and synergistic effects of phytochemicals in fruit and vegetables are responsible for their potent antioxidant and anticancer activities.

(*RH Lui, Department of Food Science, Corness University, 2003.*)

The main mechanism of cancer is damage to the DNA, where genes may mutate, and to the cell membrane, where communication takes place. These changes may trigger uncontrollable growth in cells that may then become cancerous. Cells are constantly being exposed to attack by the free radicals, or ROS, as described above. The DNA of each cell is likely attacked over 10,000 times per day, according to Dr. Bruce Ames from UC at Berkeley.

The body has repair mechanisms to cope with these problems. These mechanisms are fueled by antioxidants and anti-inflammatory micronutrients. If these nutrients are not available in adequate numbers, cancer and premature aging are likely to result. Consequently, improving our body's antioxidant defenses is absolutely essential to slowing the buildup of oxidative damage that can cause cancer and many other chronic conditions.

As we age, our chances of getting cancer increase:

	Birth-39	**40-59**	**60-79**
Male	1/60	1/12	1/3
Female	1/52	1/11	1/5

Again, the greatest factor for accelerating cancer and aging is food. Diet can impact cancer rates by an estimated 40 to 60 percent. Fruits and vegetables, the foods with the highest levels of antioxidants have been shown to decrease our chances of getting cancer and premature aging.

Toxic environments, where exposure to heavy metals, pesticides, plastics, dioxins, chlorinated agents, etc, trigger mutations in DNA and cell membranes, causing cancer directly. They also act like free radicals that need to be neutralized by our body stores of antioxidants. Consequently, the more toxins in the environment, the more we use up these micronutrients to protect ourselves. Eventually we may not have enough antioxidants to detoxify these compounds. This leads to higher risks of mutations.

Because Ningxia wolfberry fruit exerts liver protection and anti-cancer effects at the same time, some scientists believe that the fruit may be a good supplement for preventing liver cancer. Studies have shown that wolfberry led to a regression of cancer in 75 percent of patients. Other studies have shown that wolfberries can increase the sensitivity to radiation therapy and enhance the immune system of cancer patients.

The micronutrients found in wolfberry have also been found to be the most potent to counteract mutations leading to cancer. In addition, the ingredients added to wolfberry to create wolfberry juice, like pomegranate, have also been shown to reduce our risk of getting cancer. Limonene from oranges, another ingredient of wolfberry juice, has also been shown to reduce our risk of cancer. In a University of Wisconsin study, a diet with just 1% of Limonene reduced tumor counts by 25%. It was found that the main mechanism of anticancer action of limonene was to increase levels of the master antioxidant, glutathione.

RESEARCH EVIDENCE

- "A study of the anti-cancer effect of Ningxia Wolfberry,"
  J. Traditional Chinese Medicine 1989;9:117.
- "Observation of the effects of cancer therapy combined with Lycium barbarum polysaccharides in the treatment of 75 cancer patients,"
  J. Zhonghua Zhong Liu Za Zhi 1994;16:428.
- "Advances in Immuno-pharmacology study of Lycium barbarum," J. Zhon Yao Cai 2000;23:295.
- "Effect of pure and crude Lycium barbarum polysaccharides on Immuno-pharmacology,"
  J. Zhong Yao Cai 1999;22:246.
- "Inhibition of growth of human leukemia cells by Lycium barbarum polysaccharide,"
  J. Wei Sheng Yan Jiu 2001;30:333.
- "The inhibitory effect of extracts of Fructus lycii on DNA breakage by alternariol,"
  J. Biomedical Environmental Science 1996;9:67.

Polyphenols — American J. Clinical Nutrition supp 2005;81#1 .
Ellagic acid — J. Teratology 1992;46:109.
Pycnogenol — J. Agricultural Food Chemistry 2000;48:5630.
Quercetin — J. Agricultural Food Chemistry 1999;47:397.
Polysaccharides — J. Zhingghua Zhong Liu Za Zhi 1994;16:303.
Anthocyanidins — J. Biophysical research Communication 1995;214:755.

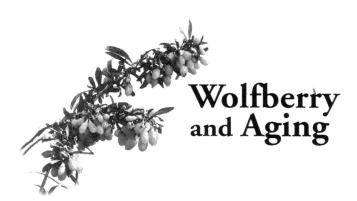

Wolfberry and Aging

It is not uncommon to find people living productive lives well beyond 100 years in Ningxia, China. Dr. Shengyuan Lei who is 103 years old takes a daily three-mile trek before he spends an hour in meditation and yoga. After this daily routine he begins to see his patients. Ma Wangshi enjoys working in her garden daily. She is 121 years old. The Hongzhangs, both 110 years of age, still enjoy shopping at the market.

All of these individuals believe that eating wolfberries daily is the most important factor in their exceptional health and longevity. The elderly in Ningxia attribute their good health and vitality to wolfberries. A bowl of fresh wolfberries every day is a part of life. Stories of the berries' health benefits have been handed down for generations. Today the wolfberry is regarded as a national treasure.

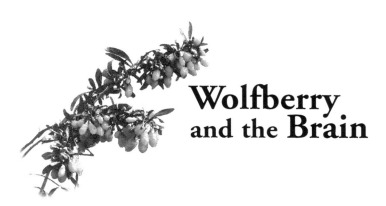

Wolfberry
and the Brain

Brain cells are the same as any other cell. Consequently they work through the same 4 mechanisms of cell membrane function, and through the Psycho-Neuro-Immune-Endocrine system of cell communication. Once this simple concept is understood, the importance of micronutrients, specifically those found in wolfberry does not need to be repeated: these mechanisms work on every organ system.

RESEARCH EVIDENCE

- "Antioxidant-rich diets improve cerebellar physiology and motor learning in aged rats," J. Brain Research 2000;866:211 (study of berries, in general).
- "Reversals of age-related declines in neuronal signal transduction, cognitive, and motor behavioral deficits with blueberry, spinach, or strawberry dietary supplementation," J. Neuroscience 1999;19:8114 (these foods raised Glutathione levels).

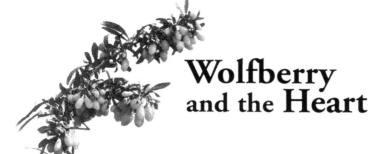

Wolfberry
and the Heart

The cells lining the arteries are called "endothelium." We now know that this is where heart disease starts. The cell membranes lining arterial walls may suffer from a lack of antioxidants, anti-inflammatory micronutrients, good sugars (polysaccharides,) lack of energy within themselves and toxins. These problems cause the endothelium to secrete substances that lead to sticky and leaky blood vessels and clotting and spasms of the muscles lining the arteries. These events lead to hypertension, plaque formation and clotting, with resulting lack of circulation throughout the body, not just the heart.

Studies have shown that oxidative stress is the unifying mechanism for atherosclerosis and hypertension. Inflammation, refined sugar toxicity, and mitochondrial dysfunction also contribute. As expected, a high antioxidant diet including fruits like the wolfberry will prevent these problems years before plaque forms in arteries and before blood pressure goes up. Further studies have shown that wolfberry can increase the function of the heart muscle and reduce blood pressure.

RESEARCH EVIDENCE

- "Dietary antioxidant flavonoids and risk of coronary heart disease," J. Lancet 1993;342:1007 (Study of Quercetin, found in Wolfberry).
- "The effects of Lycium barbarum polysaccharide on vascular tension in two-kidney one clip model of hypertension,"
  J. Sheng Li Xue Bao 1998;50:309.
- "Studies on the glycoconjugates and glycans (polysaccharides) from Lycium barbarum in inhibiting LDL peroxidation," J. Xao Xue Bao 2001;36:108.
- "Combination Fructus Lycii tablets in the treatment of hyperlipidemia,"
  J. Traditional Chinese Medicine 1995;15:178 (LDL lowered 87%).

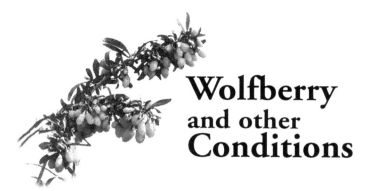

Wolfberry and other Conditions

Once we strike at the root of problems, as outlined above, it is fairly easy to see why wolfberry has salutary effects on every other organ system.

Anciently wolfberry was used for many different conditions. It was thought to have a positive effect on the liver and kidneys. It was also used for low-grade abdominal pain and to cure bed-wetting. Wolfberries were thought to be effective for those who suffered from diabetes in helping to regulate blood sugar levels. It was used to cure impotence in the reproductive system for men. Another of its functions was a tonic for the eyes, and it was well known for improving eye conditions. The wolfberry helped with dizziness, blurred vision and diminished sight. It strengthened the respiratory system and was useful in conditions with a consumptive cough. It also was known to increase immunity. The berry was known to help maintain overall health for those who suffered from chronic conditions. It was used for headaches and insomnia. Today wolfberries are known to reduce fever, sweating, irritability and thirst. They can also help stop nosebleeds, reduce vomiting and soothe coughs and wheezing.

RESEARCH EVIDENCE

- "Pregnancy in premature ovarian failure after therapy using Wolfberry (plus other antioxidants,)"
  J. Chang Gung Medicine 2003;26:449.
- "Hepatoprotective pyrrole derivatives of Lycium chinense fruits," J. Bioorganic Medicine & Chemistry 2003;13:79.
- "LCC, a crebroside from Lycium chinense, protects cultured rat hepatocytes exposed to galactosamine,"
  J. Phytotherapy Research 2000;14:448.
- "Biologic mechanism of the protective role of Lutein and Zeaxanthin (found in Wolfberry) in the eye,"
  J. Annual Review of Nutrition 2003;23:171.
- "The effect of Lycium barbarum on antioxidant activity in the retina of diabetic rats,"
  www.richnature.com
  http://www.mdidea.com/products/herbextract/wolfberry/data.html

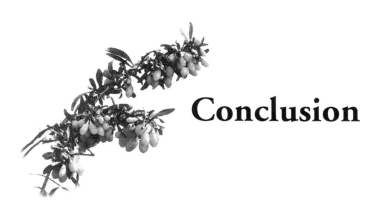

Conclusion

Wolfberry has micronutrients that work on the very common denominators of health and disease. In addition, wolfberry juice has ingredients that add even more of these micronutrients, which make our cell membranes very flexible and receptive to all messengers of cell communication. The end result is a significant improvement on how our cells work together.

Antioxidant and anti-inflammatory micronutrients keep our cell membranes from oxidizing and becoming inflamed. They also improve our detoxification pathways, so that we can get rid of toxins from the environment that act as ROS, further increasing cell membrane oxidation/inflammation and toxicity, if they are not eliminated and neutralized in a timely fashion. Ningxia wolfberry contains the highest natural amounts of important and rare antioxidants and sugars. Ounce for ounce it may be the most nutrient dense food on the planet. The wolfberry also has powerful immune-supporting agents.

The role of polysaccharides, or good sugars found in wolfberry must be re-emphasized: We noted above that one of the most toxic substances in our environment is refined sugar. It poisons our cell membranes, creating practically all types of diseases. This is a simple concept to understand, once we see that cell membrane receptors are really glycoproteins, or proteins that are not going to function, or properly construct, if they do not get the right sugars (polysaccharides) from our diets.

Since the intestines contain 60% of the immune system, 95% of neurotransmitters, and many hormones, it follows that the health of our intestines is vital in maintaining health throughout our bodies. This is why "food is the best medicine." Consequently, a diet high in antioxidants, correct sugars (polysaccharides) and fiber, such as provided by Ningxia Wolfberries, is going to provide excellent support for our intestinal functions.

Many keys to long life, health, energy and vitality can be found in the tiny red fruit known as the Ningxia wolfberry. Today this gift from the beautiful Ningxia region, also known as "China's herbal medicine valley," has been combined with a synergistic blend of fruits and is now available as a juice that offers longevity and vitality. Wolfberry juice continues a long tradition of optimal health by making the "red diamond" berry from the Ningxia province available to people all over the world.

REFERENCES CITED

Introduction
- "Nutrition Guidance of Family Doctors towards best practice," Proceedings of the Third Heelsum International Workshop, Netherlands, December 2001; American Journal of Clinical Nutrition 2003;77:1001S.
- "What is nutrition?" American Journal of Clinical Nutrition 2003;77:149.
- "We hate big pharma but we sure love drugs," December 27th, 2004, page 56.
- "Crossing the quality chasm: a new health care system for the 21st century," Institute of Medicine, 2001
- "Critical condition: how health care in America became big business and bad medicine," by Bartlett and Steele, Pulitzer Prize winners form the New York Times. J. Science 2002;296:698.
- "Critical condition: how health care in America became big business and bad medicine," by Bartlett and Steele, Pulitzer Prize winners form the New York Times. J. Science 2002;296:698.
- "The puzzle of complex diseases," The journal Science 2002;296:605 J. Immunology Today 1994;15:504.
  Journal of the American Medical Association 2004;291:358.

Basic Mechanisms of Disease
- Journal of the American Medical Association 2004;291:358. It is on *"Neuroprotection in Parkinson's Disease,"*
- New England Journal of Medicine 2000;343:78.
- Science 2002;296:605 *"The puzzle of complex diseases,"*
- The journal of the American Medical Association 2001;286:327 *"CRP, Interleukin 6, and Risk of Developing Type 2 Diabetes Mellitus."*
- J. Science 2003;300:1527.
- J. Current Opinion Clinical Nutrition Metabolic Care 2002;5:551.
- J. Circulation 2004;110:380.
- JAMA 2000;283:2235.
- J. Arteriosclerosis, Thrombosis and Vascular Biology 2003;23:1042, JAMA 2003;289:1799, J. FASEB 2004;18:1657.
- J. Family Practice News, March 2004, p11.
- J. Lancet 1996;347:949.
- J. Diabetes Care 2000;23:1278,
- J. Circulation 2003;107:1448.
- J. Artherosclerosis Thrombosis and Vascular Biology 2001;21:881.
- J. Endocrine Reviews 2003;24:278
- J. Circulation 2004;109:2
- Am J Clin Nut 2002;75:492
- Am J. Med 2002;112:275.
- J. Free Radical Biol Med 2001;31:53.

- J. Endocrine Reviews 2004;25:612.
- J. Arteriosclerosis Thrombosis Vascular Biology 2004;24:823,
- J. Faseb 2003;17:127
- J. Science 2002;298:2149
- J. Internal Med 2002;251:69, J. Diabetologia 2004;47:794.
- British J. Nutrition 2002;87:227.
- New England J. of Medicine 2001;345:1772.
- JAMA 2004;292:2823
- J. Metabolism 2001;50:868.
- European J. Clin Nut 2002;56:1137.
- NEJM 2003;348:2656
- JAMA 2004;291:679.
- J. Biol Chem 2003;278:5828.
- NEJM 2004;350:664.
- J. Environmental Health Perspectives 2003;111:a376
- J. Science 2002;297:1795.
- J. Glycoscience and Nutrition 2001;2#14.
- (J. Glycobiology 1998;8:285.)
- J. Biochimie 1998;80:75.
- J. Scientific American, July 2002, p40.
- J. Acta Anatomica 1998;161:1.
- J. BioTechnology 1990;8:108.

Wolfberry
See pesticide, fertilizer and food additives application files:
- NY/T392-2000, NY/T393-2000 and NY/T394-2000.
- *Free Radicals in Biology and Medicine*, 3rd edition, Oxford University Press, 1998 USDA 1999.
- J. National Cancer Institute 2003;95:346.

Wolfberry Cancer
- New England Journal of medicine 2003;139:51.
- RH Lui, Department of Food Science, Cornell University, 2003.
- *"Membrane and receptor modifications of oxidative stress vulnerability in aging. Nutritional considerations."* J. Annals of the New York Academy of Science 1998;854:268.
- J. Pharmacology Toxicology 1993;72:116.
- J. Food Chemical Toxicology 1998;36:637.

Wolfberry and the Brain
- J. Brain Research 2000;866:211
- J. Neuroscience 1999;19:8114

Wolfberry and the Heart
- J. Atherosclerosis Thrombosis Vascular Biology 2005;25:29.
- New England Journal of Medicine 2004;350:5,
- J. Free Radical Biology Medicine 2001;31:53.
- J. Lancet 1993;342:1007
- J. Sheng Li Xue Bao 1998;50:309
- J. Xao Xue Bao 2001;36:108
- J. Traditional Chinese Medicine 1995;15:178

Wolfberry and other Conditions
- J. Chang Gung Medicine 2003;26:449
- J. Bioorganic Medicine & Chemistry 2003;13:79
- J. Phytotherapy Research 2000;14:448
- J. Annual Review of Nutrition 2003;23:171
  http://www.chinadaily.com.cn/chinagate/doc/2004-07/19/content_349679.htm
  http://www.naturalhealthway.com/wolfberry/wolberrystudies/wolberrystudies.html

Made in the USA
San Bernardino, CA
08 July 2017